The Ketogenic Diet Guide

Including a Diet Guide and 25 Delicious
Recipes

Copyright © 2015, Heather Wedert

All rights Reserved. No part of this publication or the information in it may be quoted from or reproduced in any form by means such as printing, scanning, photocopying or otherwise without prior written permission of the copyright holder.

Disclaimer and Terms of Use:

Effort has been made to ensure that the information in this book is accurate and complete, however, the author and the publisher do not warrant the accuracy of the information, text and graphics contained within the book due to the rapidly changing nature of science, research, known and unknown facts and internet. The Author and the publisher do not hold any responsibility for errors, omissions or contrary interpretation of the subject matter herein. This book is presented solely for motivational and informational purposes only.

Table of Contents

Introduction

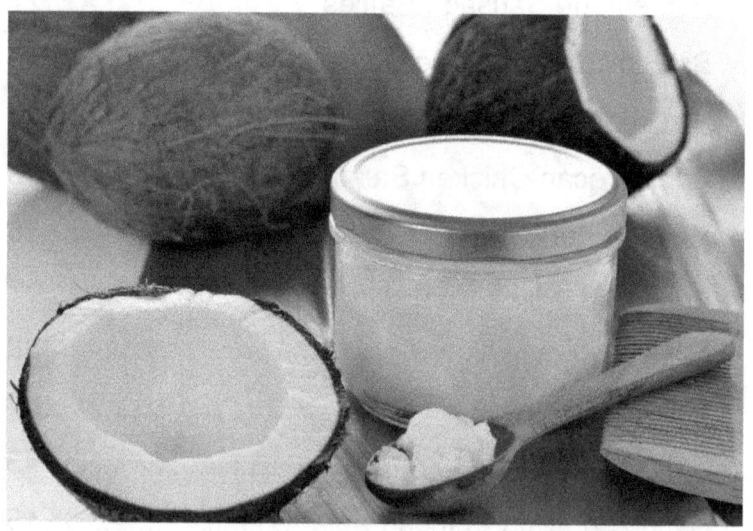

There are countless fad diets out there
promising unrealistic weight loss results or magical

relief from chronic diseases. While many of those diets do not live up to their lofty promises, the Ketogenic Diet does exactly what it says it will. The Ketogenic Diet is a high-fat, low-carbohydrate diet that not only helps you to lose weight but it is also a dietary treatment for epilepsy. The goal of this diet is to change your eating habits, reducing your consumption of carbohydrates and increasing your consumption of fats so that your body switches over to burning fat as fuel. If you think that the Ketogenic Diet might be right for you, this book is the perfect place for you to start. In this book you will receive an introduction to the Ketogenic Diet as well as an overview of the diet's restrictions. You will also find a collection of 25 delicious Ketogenic Diet recipes to help you get started on the diet. So what are you waiting for, get cooking!

About the Ketogenic Diet

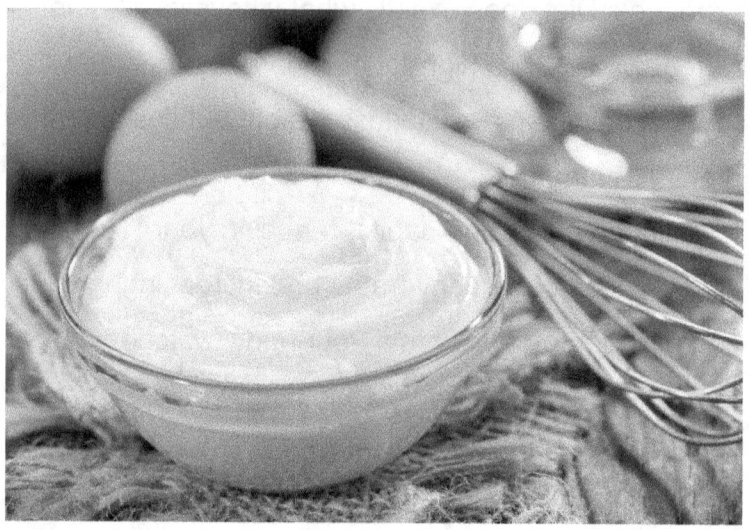

The Ketogenic Diet is an excellent tool for weight loss, especially if you have stubborn belly fat. Many people who try to lose weight find it difficult to shed fat from their bellies but, with the Ketogenic Diet, it is easy. The idea behind the Ketogenic Diet is that, by reducing your intake of carbohydrates and increasing your intake of fats, your body will go into a state of ketosis and start burning fat for fuel. Normally your body uses glucose as its primary form of energy – carbs are digested and burned for fuel almost as quickly as you eat them while fats are sometimes stored, especially in the stomach, thighs and buttocks. If you reduce your intake of carbohydrates your body will have less glucose available and, as a result, it will start burning fats – this is what it means when your body goes into a state of ketosis.

In order to adhere to the rules of the Ketogenic Diet you should restrict your carbohydrate consumption to between 20 and 60 grams per day. The amount of protein and fat you eat will depend on your size, sex and activity level but you should aim for about 70 to 75% of your daily calories from fat, 20% from protein, and the rest from carbohydrates. Below you will find a list of foods to avoid on the Ketogenic Diet as well as a list of approved foods:

Foods to Avoid

- Wheat
- Barley
- Rye
- Triticale
- Corn
- Millet
- Bulgur
- Sorghum
- Rice
- Amaranth
- Buckwheat
- Quinoa

- Couscous
- Bread
- Pasta
- Sugar
- Agave
- Processed foods
- Artificial sweetener
- Canola oil
- Corn oil
- Vegetable oils
- Low-fat foods
- Low-carb foods
- Milk
- Pineapple
- Mango
- Banana
- Papaya
- Tangerine
- Grapes
- Dried fruit
- Soy products

Foods to Enjoy Freely

- Avocado
- Butter
- Ghee
- Tallow
- Olive oil
- Coconut oil
- Coconut butter
- Palm oil

- Peanut butter
- Mayonnaise
- Grass-fed meat
- Fish and shellfish
- Eggs
- Poultry
- Bacon and sausage
- Spinach
- Kale
- Lettuce
- Radishes
- Celery
- Asparagus
- Cucumber
- Squash
- Zucchini
- Spaghetti squash
- Coconut
- Macadamia nuts
- Mayonnaise
- Mustard
- Pesto
- Fermented foods
- Spices
- Fresh herbs
- Whey protein

Foods to Eat Occasionally

- Cabbage
- Cauliflower
- Broccoli
- Brussels sprouts
- Eggplant
- Tomatoes
- Peppers
- Leeks
- Onions
- Mushrooms
- Garlic
- Pumpkin
- Sea vegetables
- Berries
- Grain-fed meats
- Full-fat yogurt
- Cottage cheese
- Sour cream
- Full-fat cheese
- Bacon
- Nuts and seeds
- Fermented soy products
- Carrot
- Sweet potato
- Parsnips
- Watermelon
- Honeydew
- Peaches
- Nectarine
- Apple
- Grapefruit

- Kiwi
- Oranges
- Cherries
- Plums
- Dried fruit

- Wine
- Cocoa powder
- Arrowroot powder

- Stevia
- Dark chocolate

Many people who hear about the Ketogenic Diet think that it will not work because eating fat will make you fat. In reality, the only thing that truly matters is that you are consuming fewer calories than you burn each day. The type of calories you consume also makes a difference, especially if you are trying to make sure that the extra calories your body burns come from stored fat. The Ketogenic Diet is not meant to be complicated and you do not need to eat any special foods – you simply have to follow the basic rules that have already been outlined for you. One thing you need to keep in mind before switching to this diet is that high-fat diets may not be healthy for individuals with certain health conditions like pancreatitis, gall bladder disease, liver disease, or kidney failure. Consult your physician before switching to the Ketogenic Diet to make sure it is the right diet for you.

Ketogenic Diet Recipes

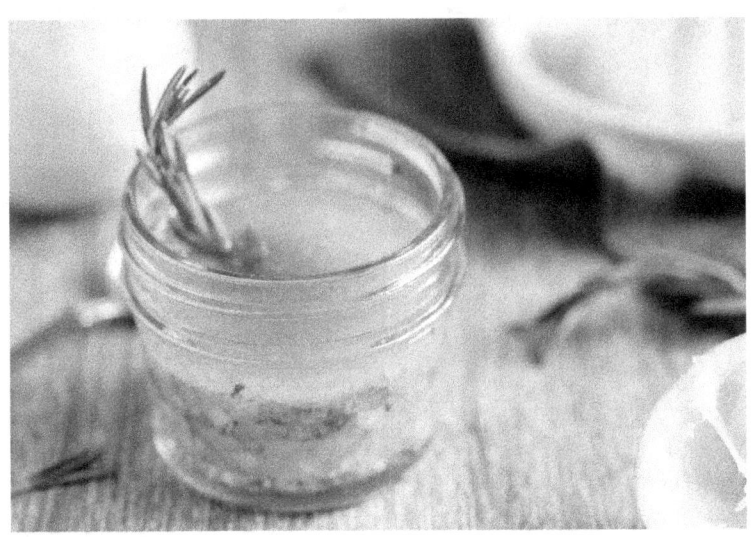

Recipes Included in this Book:

Ham and Cheese Egg Cups

Avocado Walnut Smoothie

Coconut Flour Waffles

Eggs Baked in Avocado

Cinnamon Blueberry Pancakes

Peanut Butter Banana Smoothie

Homemade Sausage Patties

Broccoli Cheddar Egg Cups

Greek Yogurt Blackberry Smoothie

Apple Pecan Chicken Salad

Hearty Beef Vegetable Stew

Easy Egg Salad

Spicy Cabbage Soup

Greek-Style Tuna Salad

Split Pea and Ham Soup

Bacon and Egg Spinach Salad

Authentic Egg Drop Soup

Rosemary Roasted Lamb Chops

Balsamic Grilled Salmon

Blue Cheese Turkey Burgers

Bacon-Wrapped Chicken Tenders

Parmesan-Crusted Tilapia

Vanilla Frozen Yogurt

Chocolate Coconut Cupcakes

Chocolate Chia Pudding

Ham and Cheese Egg Cups

Servings: 12

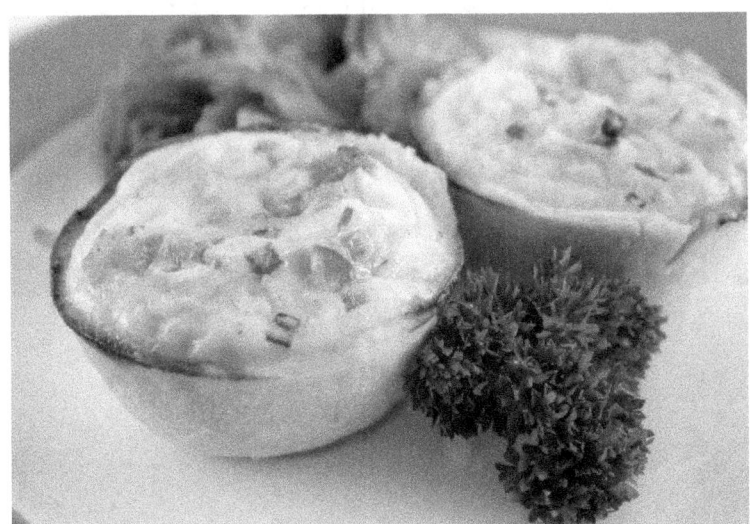

Ingredients:

12 large eggs, whisked

½ teaspoon salt

¼ teaspoon black pepper

½ cup shredded cheese (your choice)

½ lbs. diced ham

Instructions:

1. Preheat the oven to 350°F (180 C) and grease a muffin pan with cooking spray.
2. Combine the eggs, salt, pepper and cheese in a mixing bowl.
3. Divide the ham among the muffin tin cups.

4. Pour in the egg mixture, filling the cups almost full.
5. Bake for 20 to 25 minutes until the egg is set.

Avocado Walnut Smoothie

Servings: 1 to 2

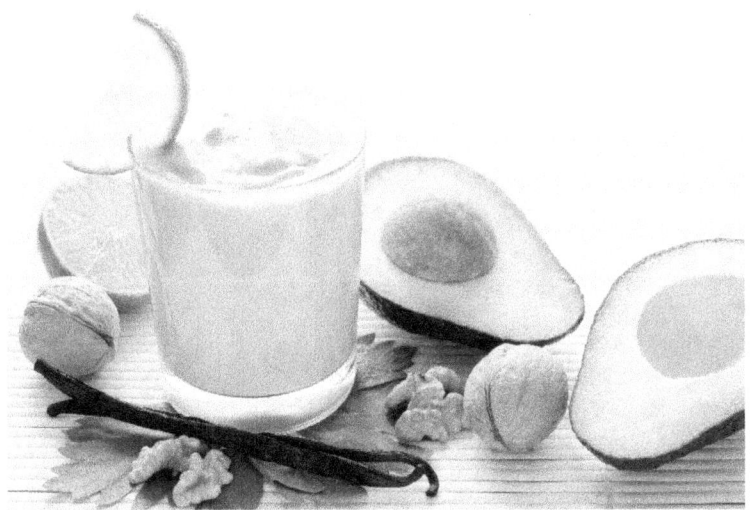

Ingredients:

1 medium ripe avocado, pitted and chopped

1 small frozen banana, peeled and sliced

1 cup unsweetened almond milk

½ cup ice cubes

2 tablespoons chopped walnuts

2 tablespoons fresh lime juice

Instructions:

1. Combine the ingredients in a high-speed blender.

2. Blend the mixture for 30 to 60 seconds until smooth and well combined.
3. Divide the smoothie between two glasses and enjoy immediately.

Coconut Flour Waffles

Servings: 4

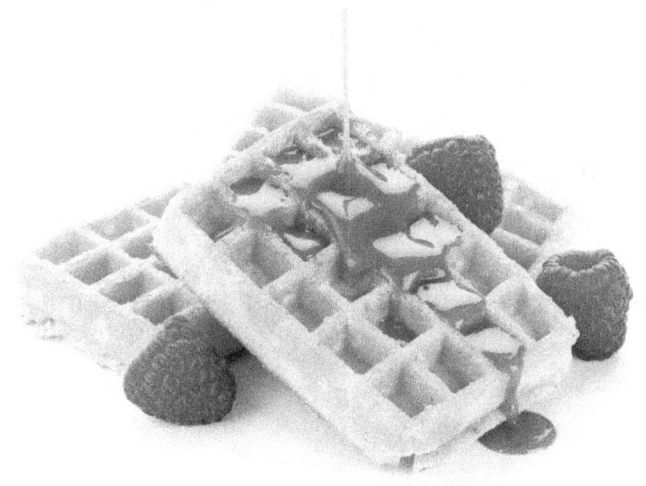

Ingredients:

½ cup coconut flour

½ cup whey protein powder

1 cup unsweetened almond milk

3 tablespoons coconut oil, melted

4 large eggs, whisked

1 teaspoon cream of tartar

½ teaspoon baking soda

½ to 1 teaspoon liquid Stevia

Instructions:

1. Preheat a waffle iron as directed.
2. Combine the flour, protein powder, cream of tartar and baking soda in a mixing bowl.
3. In a separate bowl, whisk together the almond milk, coconut oil, eggs and stevia.
4. Whisk the dry ingredients into the wet until smooth and well combined.
5. Spoon the batter into the waffle iron and cook according to the directions.
6. Serve the waffles hot with peanut butter, if desired.

Eggs Baked in Avocado

Servings: 4

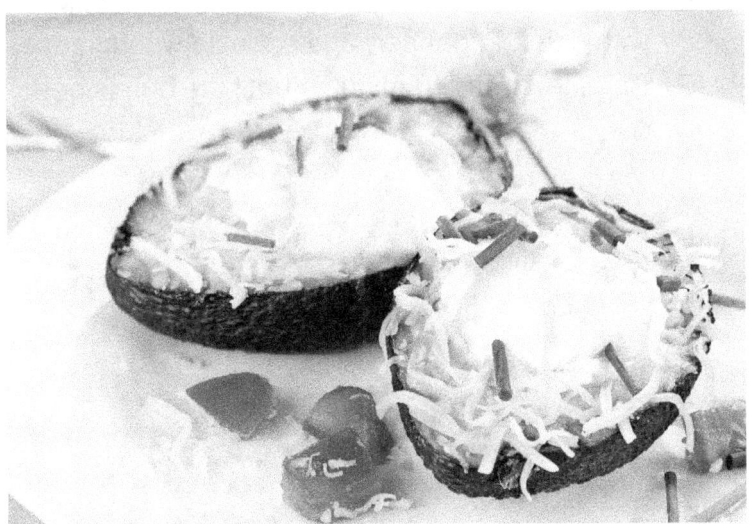

Ingredients:

2 medium ripe avocado

4 large eggs

Salt and pepper to taste

½ cup shredded cheddar cheese

Instructions:

1. Preheat the oven to 425°F and grease a baking dish with oil.
2. Cut the avocados in half and remove the pits – scoop out 2 to 3 tablespoons of avocado from each half.

3. Place the avocado halves upright in the baking dish.
4. Crack an egg into each avocado half, season with salt and pepper, and sprinkle with cheese.
5. Bake for 15 to 20 minutes until the egg is set.

Cinnamon Blueberry Pancakes

Servings: 4

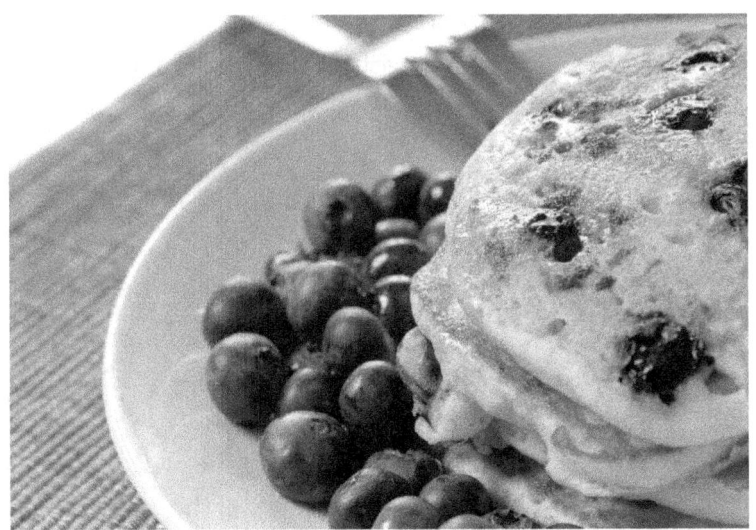

Ingredients:

1 cup almond flour

1 teaspoon ground cinnamon

1 teaspoon cream of tartar

¾ teaspoon baking soda

5 large eggs, whisked well

¼ cup coconut oil

1 tablespoons vanilla extract

1 teaspoon liquid Stevia

1 ½ cups fresh blueberries

Instructions:

1. Combine the flour, cinnamon, baking soda, cream of tartar in a mixing bowl.
2. Beat the eggs in another mixing bowl then whisk in the coconut oil, vanilla extract and Stevia.
3. Whisk the dry ingredients into the wet until smooth and well combined.
4. Preheat a large nonstick skillet over medium-high heat.
5. Spoon the batter into the skillet, using about 3 tablespoons per pancake.
6. Sprinkle a few blueberries into the wet batter and cook for 2 to 3 minutes until the underside is browned.
7. Flip the pancakes and cook for another 2 minutes or so until browned.
8. Transfer the pancakes to a plate to keep warm and repeat with the remaining batter.

Peanut Butter Banana Smoothie

Servings: 1 to 2

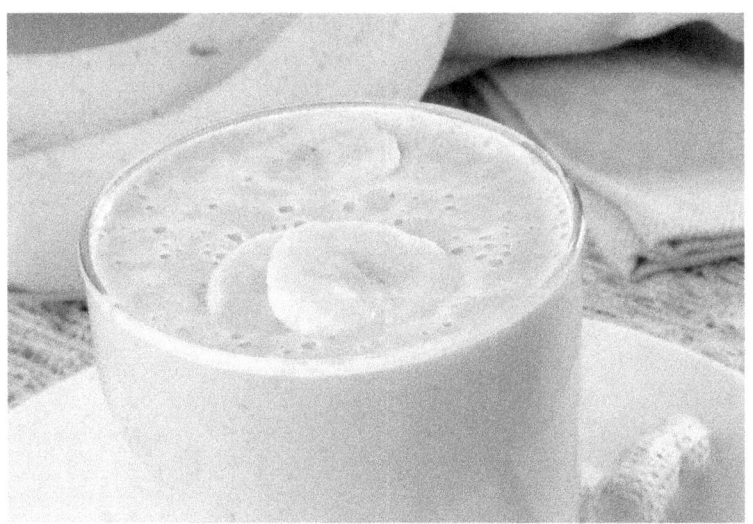

Ingredients:

2 large frozen bananas, peeled and sliced

1 cup unsweetened almond milk

½ cup plain Greek yogurt

½ cup ice cubes

2 to 3 tablespoons peanut butter

Instructions:

1. Combine the ingredients in a high-speed blender.
2. Blend the mixture for 30 to 60 seconds until smooth and well combined.

3. Divide the smoothie between two glasses and enjoy immediately.

Homemade Sausage Patties

Servings: 8

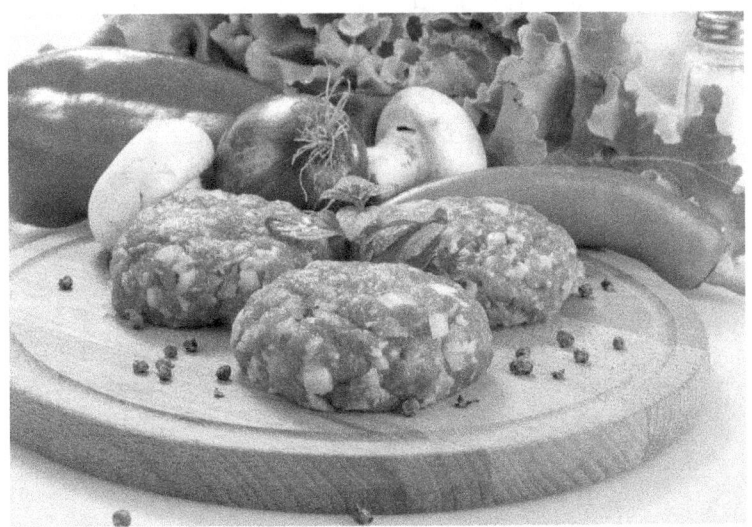

Ingredients:

1 lbs. ground pork

1 large egg, whisked

1 teaspoon minced garlic

2 teaspoons fresh chopped sage

½ teaspoon fresh chopped thyme

Salt and pepper to taste

2 teaspoons olive oil

Instructions:

1. Combine the ingredients except the oil in a large mixing bowl.

2. Stir until well combined then shape by hand into 8 even-sized patties.
3. Cover and chill for 15 minutes.
4. Preheat the oil in a large skillet over high heat.
5. Add the sausage patties and cook for 4 minutes on each side until cooked through.

Broccoli Cheddar Egg Cups

Servings: 12

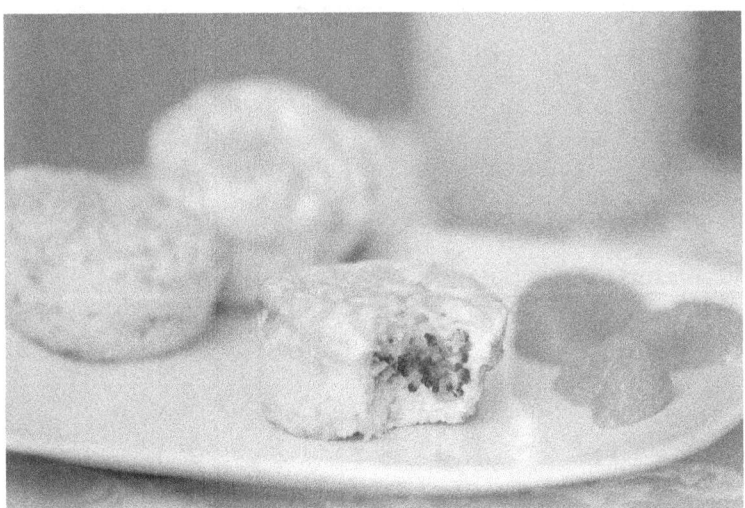

Ingredients:

12 large eggs, whisked

½ teaspoon salt

¼ teaspoon black pepper

½ cup shredded cheese (your choice)

1 ½ cups diced broccoli

Instructions:

1. Preheat the oven to 350°F and grease a muffin pan with cooking spray.
2. Combine the eggs, salt, pepper, and cheese in a mixing bowl.
3. Divide the broccoli among the muffin tin cups.

4. Pour in the egg mixture, filling the cups almost full.
5. Bake for 20 to 25 minutes until the egg is set.

Blackberry Greek Yogurt Smoothie

Servings: 1 to 2

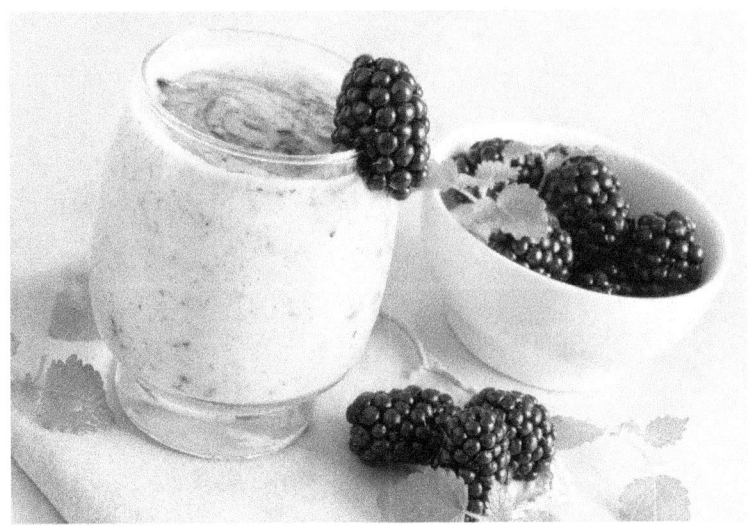

Ingredients:

1 ½ cups frozen blackberries

1 medium frozen banana, peeled and sliced

1 cup plain Greek yogurt

½ cup ice cubes

2 tablespoons fresh mint

Instructions:

1. Combine the ingredients in a high-speed blender.
2. Blend the mixture for 30 to 60 seconds until smooth and well combined.

3. Divide the smoothie between two glasses and enjoy immediately.

Apple Pecan Chicken Salad

Servings: 6

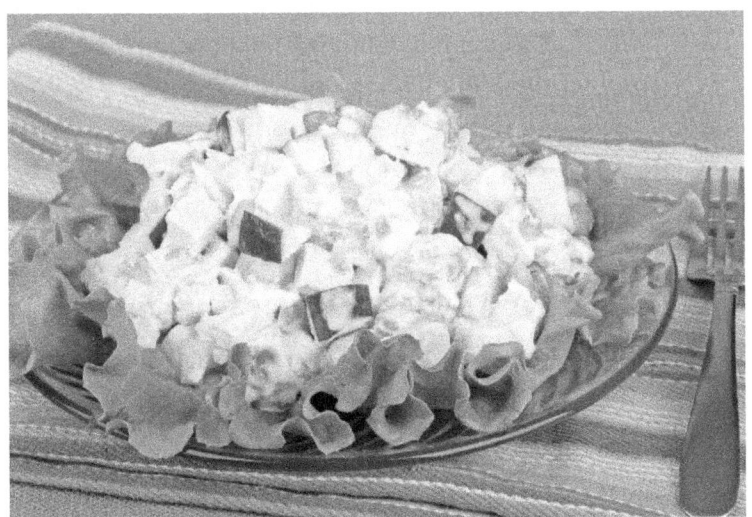

Ingredients:

½ cup mayonnaise

1/3 cup sour cream

1 teaspoon apple cider vinegar

Salt and pepper to taste

1 teaspoon fresh lemon juice

3 cups cooked chicken breast, chopped

1 large ripe apple, cored and diced

1 cup red seedless grapes, halved

1 large stalk celery, diced

¼ cup chopped pecans

Instructions:

1. Whisk together the mayonnaise, sour cream, and vinegar in a mixing bowl.
2. Season with salt and pepper to taste then whisk in the lemon juice.
3. Toss in the chicken, apples, grapes, celery and pecans.
4. Chill the salad for a few hours then serve on a bed of lettuce.

Hearty Beef Vegetable Stew

Servings: 8 to 10

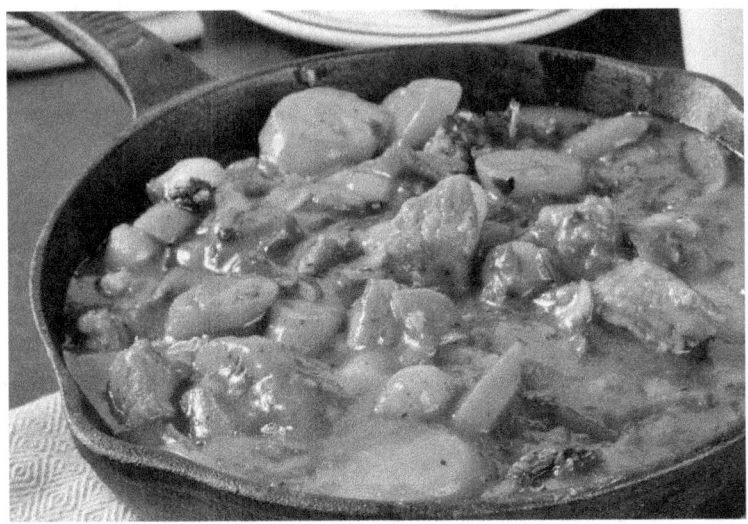

Ingredients:

1 ½ lbs. beef stew meat, cut into chunks

2 cups sliced carrots

4 medium Yukon gold potatoes, peeled and quartered

1 large yellow onion, chopped

2 stalks celery, sliced

3 cups beef broth

2 ½ tablespoons Worcestershire sauce

1 tablespoon minced garlic

Salt and pepper to taste

Instructions:

1. Combine the beef, carrots, potatoes, onion and celery in the slow cooker.
2. Whisk together the beef broth, Worcestershire sauce, garlic, salt and pepper in a small bowl.
3. Pour the mixture into the slow cooker and stir it in.
4. Cover and cook on low heat for 6 to 8 hours until the beef is cooked through.
5. Whisk together the arrowroot powder and water then stir into the slow cooker.
6. Cover and cook for 30 minutes on high heat until thickened – serve hot.

Easy Egg Salad

Servings: 4

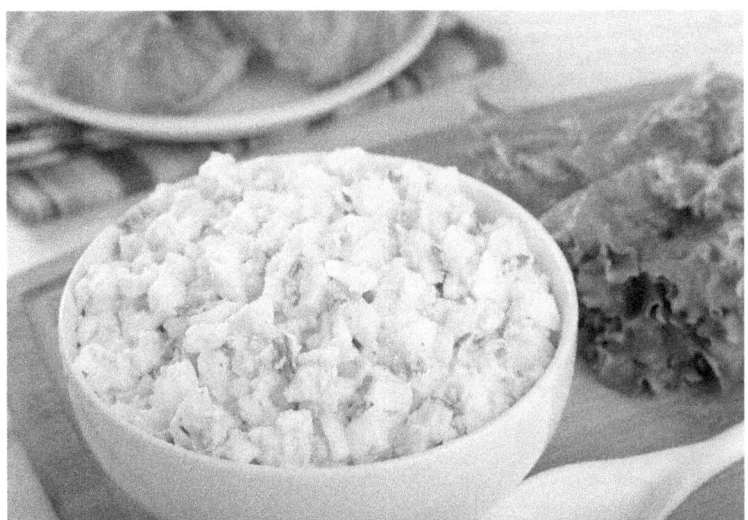

Ingredients:

4 large hardboiled eggs, peeled and chopped

¼ cup mayonnaise

½ cup diced celery

¼ cup chopped green onion

Salt and pepper to taste

Instructions:

1. Place the eggs in a large bowl and mash gently with a fork.
2. Stir in the mayonnaise, celery and onion – season with salt and pepper to taste.

3. Chill the salad until cold and serve on a bed of lettuce.

Spicy Cabbage Soup

Servings: 6 to 8

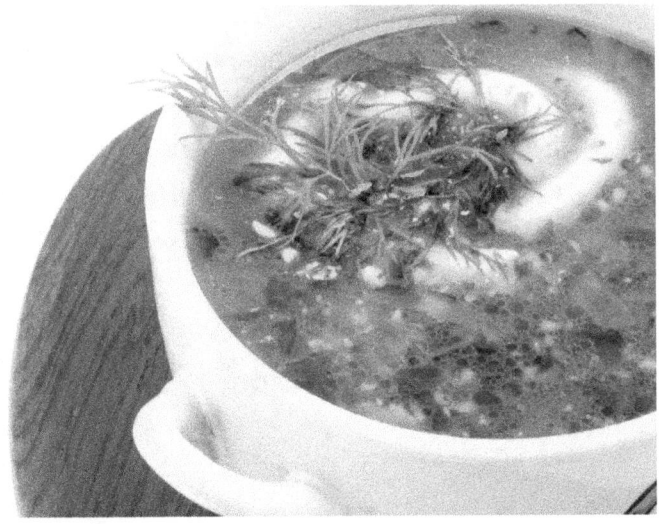

Ingredients:

1 tablespoon olive oil

1 large onion, chopped

1 tablespoon minced garlic

5 cups chicken or vegetable broth

1 small serrano pepper, seeded and minced

2 large Yukon gold potatoes, peeled and chopped

1 ½ teaspoons ground coriander

3 teaspoons dry mustard powder

3 cups sliced green cabbage

Instructions:

1. Heat the oil in a large saucepan over medium heat.
2. Add the onion and garlic then cook for 5 to 6 minutes until tender.
3. Stir in the broth, serrano pepper, potatoes, coriander and mustard.
4. Bring to a simmer and cook on low heat for 20 minutes.
5. Stir in the cabbage and cook for 5 minutes.
6. Serve hot with a dollop of sour cream.

Greek-Style Tuna Salad

Servings: 6

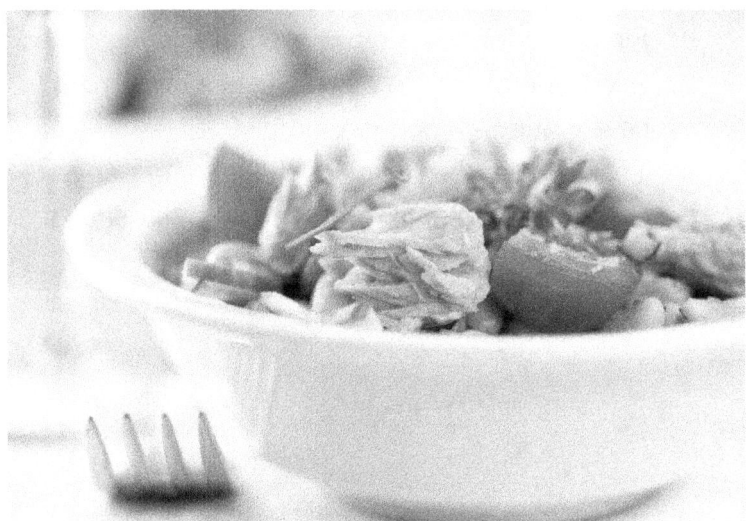

Ingredients:

3 (6-ounce) cans tuna in water, drained

1 (14 ounce) can artichoke hearts, drained and chopped

½ cup sliced black olives

½ cup chopped red onion

½ cup chopped celery

½ cup crumbled feta cheese

¼ cup olive oil

2 tablespoons white wine vinegar

Salt and pepper to taste

½ cup fresh chopped parsley

Instructions:

1. Flake the tuna into a mixing bowl.
2. Stir in the artichoke hearts, olives, red onion, celery and feta cheese.
3. Toss in the vinegar, olive oil, salt and pepper.
4. Chill the salad until ready to serve – toss in the parsley just before serving.

Split Pea and Ham Soup

Servings: 8 to 10

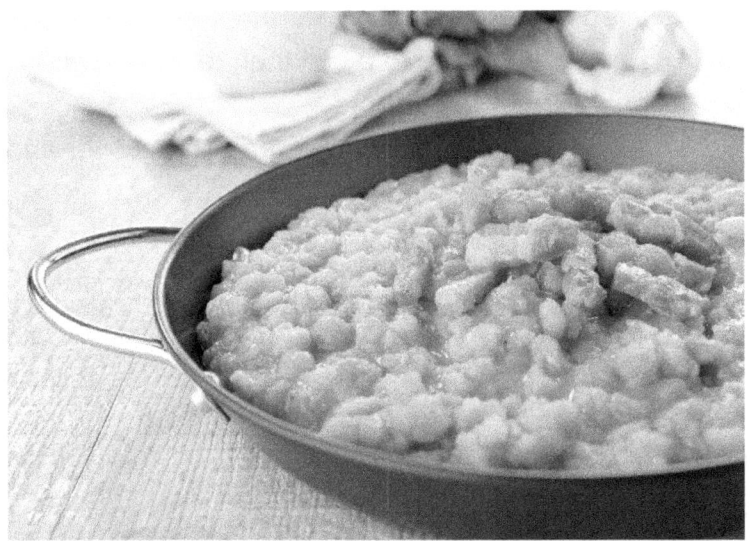

Ingredients:

2 cups dried split peas

7 cups cold water

2 cups diced cooked ham

2 cups diced baby carrots

1 cup diced yellow onion

¾ cups diced celery

1 large Yukon gold potato, peeled and diced

1 teaspoon fresh garlic, minced

Salt and pepper to taste

Instructions:

1. Combine the peas and water in a large Dutch oven over high heat.
2. Bring the mixture to a boil then reduce heat and simmer for 2 hours.
3. Stir in the remaining ingredients then cover and simmer for 30 minutes more.
4. Serve hot garnished with fresh chopped parsley.

Bacon and Egg Spinach Salad

Servings: 6

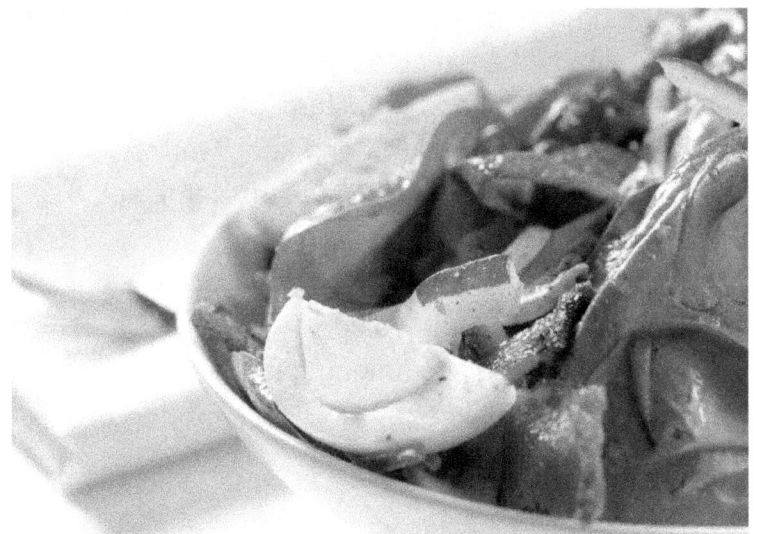

Ingredients:

10 slices bacon, chopped

¼ cup red wine vinegar

1 teaspoon Dijon mustard

5 to 10 drops liquid stevia

Salt and pepper to taste

10 ounces fresh chopped spinach

1 cup sliced mushrooms

1 small red onion, sliced thin

4 hardboiled eggs, peeled and quartered

Instructions:

1. Heat the bacon in a skillet over medium-high heat until crisp.
2. Drain the bacon on paper towels.
3. Whisk the vinegar, mustard, stevia, salt and pepper into the skillet and keep warm.
4. Place the chopped spinach in a large salad bowl.
5. Add the onion, mushrooms and cooked bacon – toss with the dressing.
6. Divide the salads among four plates and top with hardboiled egg.

Authentic Egg Drop Soup

Servings:

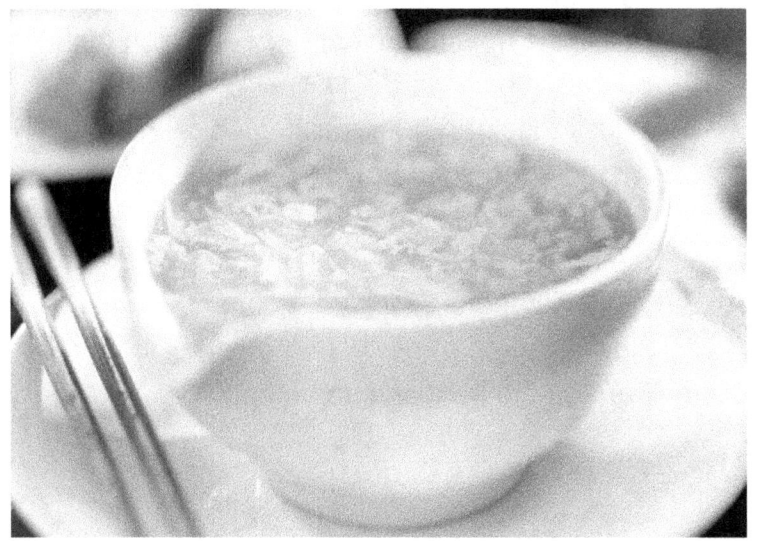

Ingredients:

4 cups chicken broth, divided

½ teaspoon fresh grated ginger

3 teaspoon soy sauce

Pinch white pepper

1 cup sliced mushrooms

2 to 3 green onions, sliced thin

1 tablespoon arrowroot powder

3 large eggs, whisked well

Instructions:

1. Whisk together 3 ½ cups chicken broth with the ginger, soy sauce and pepper in a large saucepan.
2. Stir in the mushrooms and green onion then bring to a boil.
3. Whisk together the remaining chicken broth with the arrowroot powder.
4. Stir the mixture into the saucepan and reduce the heat to a simmer.
5. While stirring the mixture, pour in the egg in a slow drizzle.
6. Turn off the heat and serve hot.

Rosemary Roasted Lamb Chops

Servings: 4 to 6

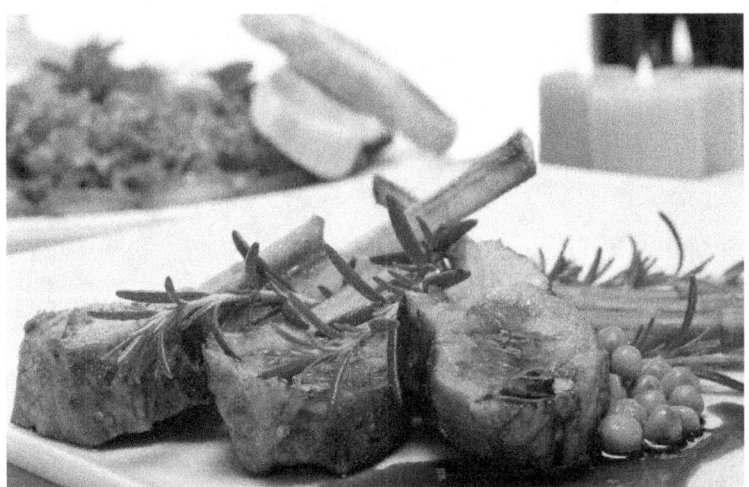

Ingredients:

2 lbs. bone-in lamb chops

1 to 2 tablespoons olive oil

Salt and pepper to taste

3 tablespoons fresh chopped rosemary

1 tablespoon fresh minced garlic

Instructions:

1. Preheat the broiler in your oven to high heat.
2. Brush the chops with olive oil and season with salt and pepper to taste.
3. Combine the rosemary and garlic in a small bowl, mashing it into a paste.

4. Arrange the lamb chops on a roaster pan and spread with the rosemary garlic paste.
5. Broil for 4 to 5 minutes on each side until cooked to the desired level.

Balsamic Grilled Salmon

Servings: 4

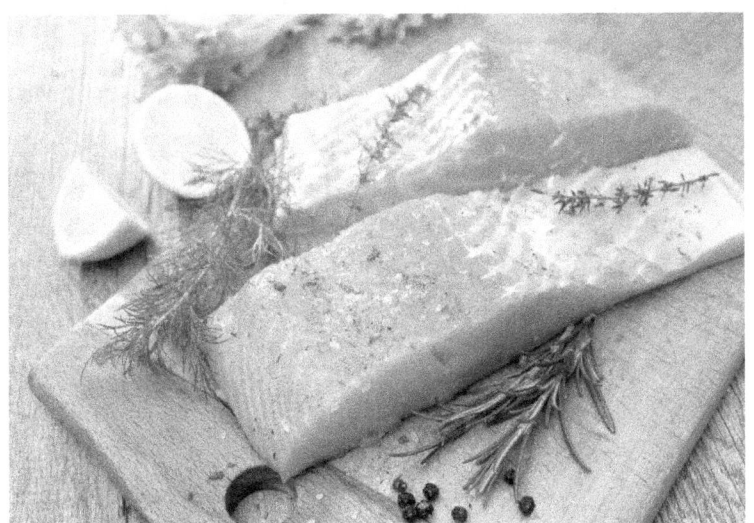

Ingredients:

¼ cup plus 2 tablespoons balsamic vinegar

¼ cup plus 2 tablespoons cooking sherry

2 tablespoons fresh lemon juice

2 tablespoons raw honey

4 (6-ounce) boneless salmon fillets

1 tablespoon olive oil

Salt and pepper to taste

Instructions:

1. Preheat the grill to medium-high heat and brush the grates with olive oil.

2. Whisk together the balsamic vinegar, sherry, lemon juice and honey in a small saucepan.
3. Bring to a simmer and cook on low heat for 15 minutes until reduced.
4. Brush the salmon with olive oil and season with salt and pepper.
5. Place the fillets on the grates and grill for 5 minutes on each side until the flesh flakes easily with a fork.
6. Serve the fillets hot drizzled with balsamic glaze.

Blue Cheese Burgers

Servings: 4

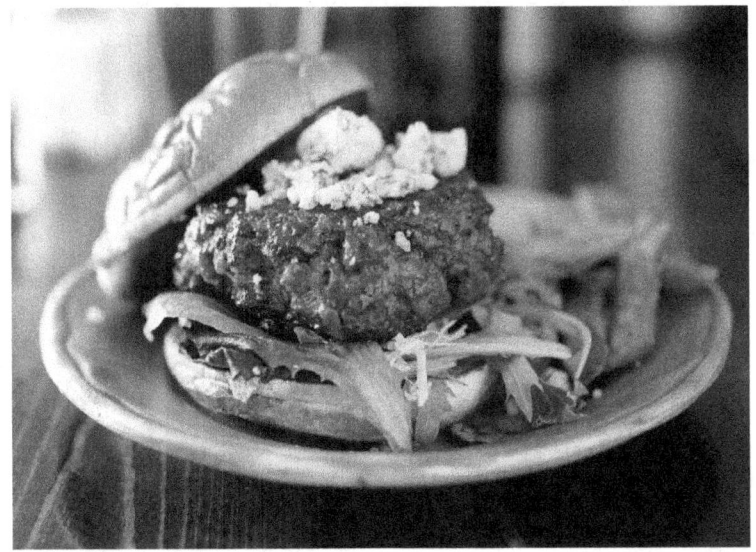

Ingredients:

1 lbs. lean ground beef

1/4 cup almond flour

2 tablespoons almond milk

½ cup blue cheese crumbles

Salt and pepper to taste

Instructions:

1. Preheat the broiler in your oven to high heat.
2. Combine all of the ingredients in a mixing bowl and stir well.

3. Shape the mixture into four even-sized patties by hand.
4. Place the patties on a roaster pan and broil for 3 to 5 minutes on each side until cooked to the desired level.

Bacon-Wrapped Chicken Tenders

Servings: 4

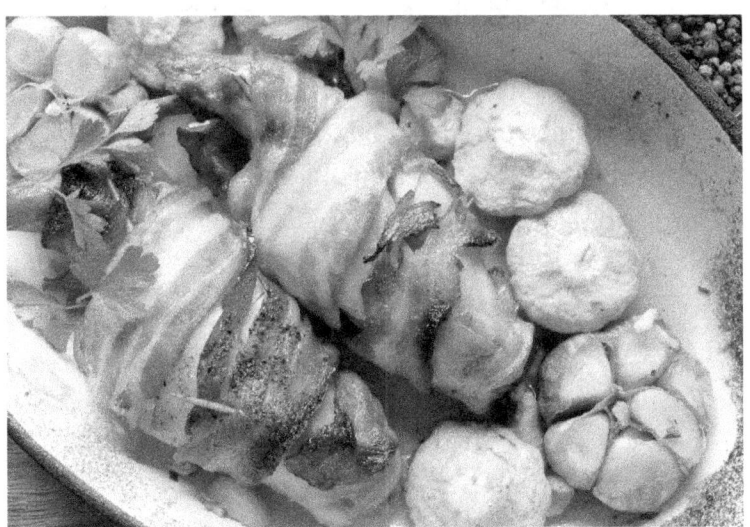

Ingredients:

1 lbs. boneless skinless chicken tenders

1 teaspoon paprika

½ teaspoon onion powder

½ teaspoon salt

¼ teaspoon black pepper

½ lbs. uncooked bacon

Instructions:

1. Preheat the oven to 350°F and line a baking sheet with foil.

2. Combine the paprika, onion powder, salt and pepper in a small bowl.
3. Sprinkle the spice mixture over the chicken tenders.
4. Wrap each tender in two slices of bacon and place them in the baking sheet.
5. Bake for 25 and 30 minutes until the chicken is cooked through.

Parmesan-Crusted Tilapia

Servings: 4

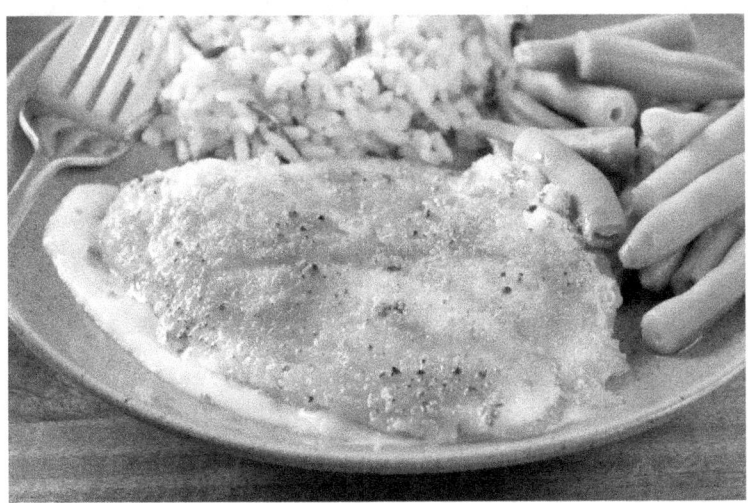

Ingredients:

4 (6-ounce) boneless tilapia fillets

2 tablespoons olive oil

Salt and pepper to taste

½ cup grated parmesan cheese

¼ cup almond flour

1 teaspoon dried parsley

Instructions:

1. Preheat the oven to 350°F and line a baking sheet with foil.
2. Brush the fillets with olive oil and season with salt and pepper to taste.

3. Combine the almond flour, parmesan cheese and parsley in a shallow dish.
4. Arrange the fillets on the baking sheet and top with the parmesan mixture.
5. Bake for 12 to 15 minutes until the flesh flakes easily with a fork.

Vanilla Frozen Yogurt

Servings: 8 to 10

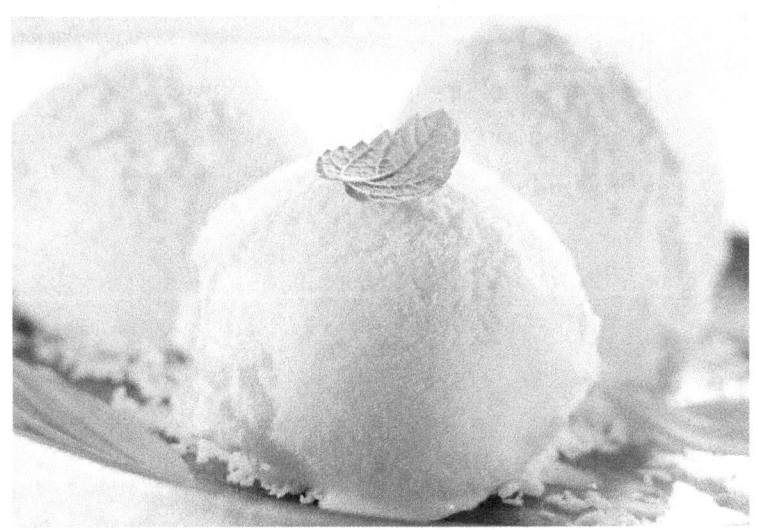

Ingredients:

2 ¼ cups heavy whipping cream

2 ¼ cups vanilla Greek yogurt

4 large egg yolks, beaten

2 ½ tablespoons vanilla extract

1 fresh vanilla bean, halved and seeds scraped

1 teaspoon liquid Stevia

1 tablespoon arrowroot powder

Instructions:

1. Beat together the cream and yogurt in a chilled bowl until soft peaks form.

2. Whisk in the egg yolks, the vanilla extract, and the vanilla bean.
3. Whisk the Stevia and arrowroot powder into the yogurt mixture.
4. Pour the mixture into an ice cream maker and freeze according to the manufacturer's directions.

Chocolate Coconut Cupcakes

Servings: 12

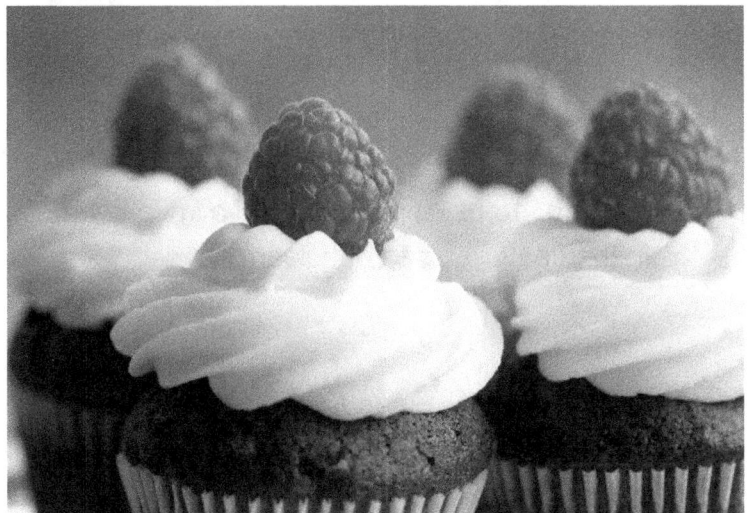

Ingredients:

1/3 cup coconut flour

1/3 cup unsweetened cocoa powder

½ teaspoon baking soda

¼ teaspoon salt

4 large eggs, whisked

½ to ¾ cup honey

½ cup unsweetened shredded coconut

Instructions:

1. Preheat the oven to 350°F (180 C) and line a muffin pan with paper liners.

2. Combine the coconut flour, cocoa powder, baking soda and salt in a mixing bowl.
3. In a separate bowl, beat together the eggs and honey then whisk in the dry ingredients until well combined.
4. Fold in the coconut then spoon the batter into the pan, filling the cups 2/3 full.
5. Bake for 18 to 20 minutes until a knife inserted in the center comes out clean.

Chocolate Chia Pudding

Servings: 4

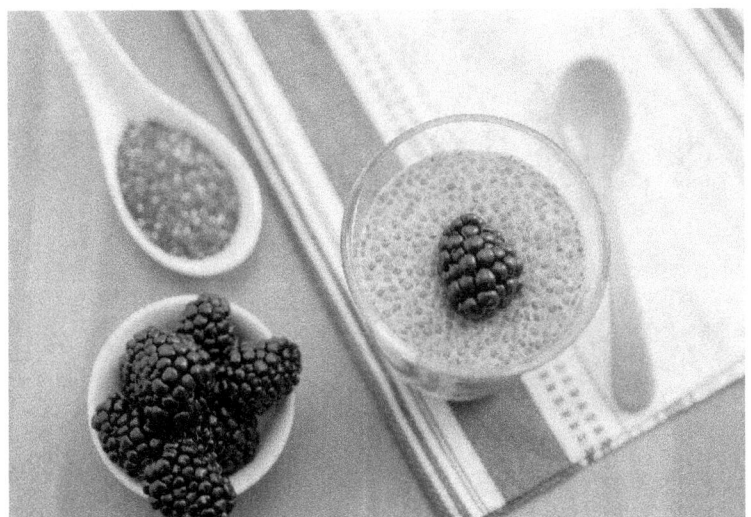

Ingredients:

1 cup chia seeds

1 cup heavy whipping cream

2 cups unsweetened almond milk

¼ cup unsweetened cocoa powder

½ to 1 teaspoon liquid Stevia

Instructions:

1. Combine the ingredients in a blender and blend smooth.
2. Divide the mixture among dessert cups.
3. Chill for at least 15 minutes before serving.

Conclusion

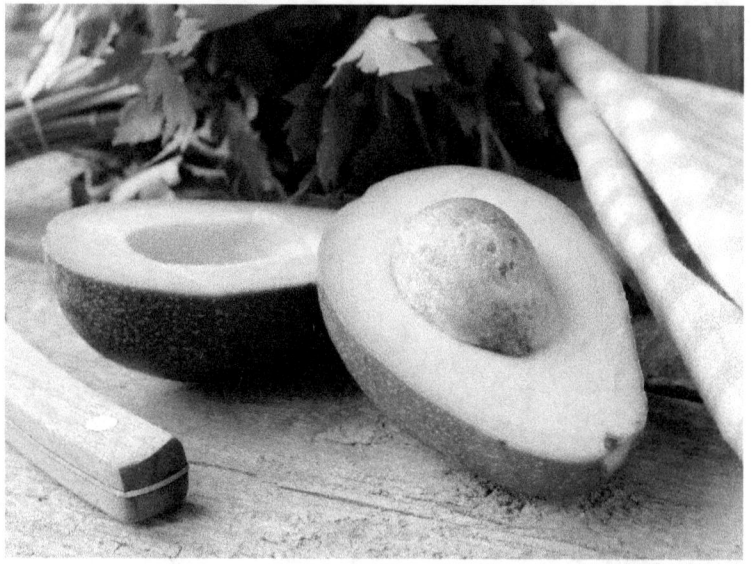

After reading this book, you should have a basic understanding of the Ketogenic Diet including a list of foods to eat and avoid. The Ketogenic Diet is an excellent tool for weight loss and many people experience additional health benefits as well. If you are ready to give the Ketogenic Diet a try this book is the perfect place to start. In addition to receive a quick-start guide to the Ketogenic Diet, you have also received a collection of delicious recipes. To get started with the Ketogenic Diet simply pick a recipe from this book and give it a try. You won't be disappointed.

www.ingramcontent.com/pod-product-compliance
Lightning Source LLC
Chambersburg PA
CBHW070324290526
45791CB00003B/1244